I0410516

SURVIVOR

My Journey Back to the Light

True Story written by Carolyn Smith

(A journey through bereavement, cancer and
resulting drug-dependency)

Dedications

Dedicated to my darling husband, Rod, my two beautiful children, Jamie and Samantha, and my sisters, Denise and Judith; without whose strength, unconditional love and unending support I would never again have reached the light.

Acknowledgements

My friend Lisa Avis, for her organisation skills.

My friend John Paul Zampetti, for his front cover design. John retains copyright for illustration.

Sandra Perry, my school saviour.

My dear stepsons, Barry and Alan.

Note for Librarians: a cataloguing record for this book that includes Dewey Classification and US Library of Congress numbers is available from the National Library of Canada. The complete cataloguing record can be obtained from the National Library's online database at:
www.nlc-bnc.ca/amicus/index-e.html
ISBN 1-4120-1952-4

TRAFFORD

This book was published on-demand in cooperation with Trafford Publishing.
On-demand publishing is a unique process and service of making a book available for retail sale to the public taking advantage of on-demand manufacturing and Internet marketing. On-demand publishing includes promotions, retail sales, manufacturing, order fulfilment, accounting and collecting royalties on behalf of the author.

Suite 6E, 2333 Government St., Victoria, B.C. V8T 4P4, CANADA
Phone 250-383-6864   Toll-free 1-888-232-4444 (Canada & US)

Fax 250-383-6804   E-mail sales@trafford.com   Web site www.trafford.com

TRAFFORD PUBLISHING IS A DIVISION OF TRAFFORD HOLDINGS LTD.

Trafford Catalogue #03-2430   www.trafford.com/robots/03-2430.html

10   9   8   7   6   5   4   3   2   1

My darling children

What incredible joy you both bring to my life.

I start my story now to help you understand how recent life events have affected me … and in turn affected you two.

Mum was diagnosed with lung cancer whilst undergoing a routine chest x-ray prior to a hip replacement. She was 59. We were completely devastated, particularly as she already had secondary tumours in the neck.

We were told that the condition was terminal with a limited prognosis of maybe six to eighteen months. Rod and I were married in August of 1994. Mum had been diagnosed in March 1994 and Dad had a leg amputated, because of coronary artery disease, in June 1994. Both were at our wedding, in body if not in mind, and Dad managed to walk me up the aisle. How much admiration I felt for them both is not possible to describe in words. Dad wept whilst attempting to make a speech. He must have felt so relieved that it was over. What a lovely day.

Mum was not offered any treatment at first, apart from resection of the neck tumours but was eventually (after months) offered chemotherapy for symptomatic relief.

Mum started to pick up. Dad got used to walking when he needed to and used an electric scooter the remainder of the time. They bought a flat near the high street and moved in late 1994. This gave them both easy access to the shops, which was an absolute must for them both. At every opportunity we treated Mum to an outing and our presents to her became lavish. Dad always chose to stay at home because his treatment didn't really allow him to wander too far from the bathroom and the fridge.

Mum remained relatively well but tired much of the time.

In October 1995 we discovered we were expecting you, darling Samantha. How much that picked up the entire family is hard to put into words, but your Nan and Grandad were given a new lease of life. Nannie got busy knitting, buying and preparing to embroider your welcome picture. I was apprehensive about your arrival because even though I was 37, I chose not to undergo any invasive tests (I didn't want to scare you by someone putting needles near to you in my tummy). But you duly arrived beautiful, healthy and safe. Daddy cried, I cried, Nannie cried and Grandad was elated. You were a difficult new baby because we never seemed to know what you wanted. I suspect I was suffering from postnatal depression and that I wasn't very good at showing you I loved you; so maybe that's why you were so upset.

I took maternity leave for six months, during which time Nannie took a turn for the worse. A tumour in her breast was irradiated, but the hospital could never conclude if it was a second primary cancer or the original primary with the lung as secondaries. She prayed the breast was the original primary because that was somehow an honourable cancer. Primaries of the lung were an old smoking man s disease. That s how Mum felt.

I returned to work with my beloved baby ensconced in a loving nursery. It was January 1997. In June, Mum was admitted as an emergency to hospital with a pleural effusion. She was a frail, pitiful sight and it nearly broke my heart. She was patched up enough to go home but needed more medication from then on. We all began to feel drained with the roller-coaster emotions. Rod and I worked all week and each weekend we were running around with Nan and Grandad, either helping them get somewhere or do something.

The Lottery Win

During these bleak times came our National Lottery win. Not the big bucks, but enough to change our level of comfort. We had such fun buying presents for everyone and clearing our numerous debts. We were able to choose instead of settling and most importantly were able to remove financial worries from our lives. A friend sent me a card saying that Christmas had come early for us that year. What an irony considering the way the real Christmas was to turn out to be.

As winter arrived so did my statutory chest infection, completely eradicating my voice.

December 1997 brought two horrors for all of us. Mum was admitted to the hospital with blood clots in the lungs that were life threatening. At the same time we were told that Rod s twin brother was undergoing some tests for acute headaches. As we had been warned not to expect Christmas with Mum, I didn t really think too deeply about my brother-in-law. Yet again Mum was patched up and sent home with oxygen. Rod went to Dorset to visit his brother on the 23rd December 1997. By now he had been admitted to hospital with a brain aneurysm. He could barely cope with the pain but knew Rod was there. On the evening of the 24th we received a phone call informing us that my brother-in-law had probably sustained brain damage after a subarachnoid haemorrhage. We wept practically all night in complete disbelief at everything we were dealing with. We tried to act normally on Christmas morning for you both but I felt ill with the chest infection and we were sick with worry over Rod s brother and Mum. Jamie my darling, you were a tower of strength through all those bleak, dark times, helping where it was possible with Samantha who we struggled to care for through our desperate pain and worry. Mum was dreadfully ill on Christmas day and we went through the farce of lunch at the local hotel. I couldn t speak at all by this stage and we had the phone switched on awaiting news from Dorset. Mum literally had to be held up on either side in order to sit up at the table. She smiled through the meal but it was only a facial expression. We don t know how she survived that day. The news we received of Rod s brother was that he continued to bleed into his brain. Rod travelled very early on Boxing morning to see him. By that evening I had been phoned by his wife to say that he was brainstem dead. I didn t even have enough voice to comfort her. I have never felt so helpless in my entire life. Strangely, although really distraught at the news about my dear brother-in-law, Mum seemed to pick up a bit after that. Where there s life, there s hope, she said and continued to smile. Losing my brother-in-law at 32 was such a tragedy and had a profound effect on Rod, and me too really. Life became so dark and bleak but still we had to keep on going because Mum and Dad increasingly needed us for company. Mum was virtually house-ridden and Dad was desperate for company on Saturday mornings for drinks and eats. So the routine was Saturday morning with Dad and Sunday morning visiting Mum and

Dad. We adored them but we were so exhausted. No time seemed to be ours. Jamie, you were such a joy to them and never gave them a hint that you were fed up at being summoned for help. Sam, you filled Nan s breaking heart and restored Grandad s laughter. What perfect grandchildren you were to them.

In May, the hospital had handed Mum to the hospice for palliative care only. This had a devastating effect on all of us, but still Mum pretended that all was fine. Dad cried a lot on Saturdays and wore himself out driving all around town buying delicious delicacies to try and tempt her appetite. The weight was dropping off her in stones. I felt so helpless and upset and angry. It had been an unreal situation ever since the diagnosis but now the roles were reversed and I felt like I was caring for my two sick children. I was in a state of mourning each day and I found it very difficult to be a working Mum whilst living through the horror of the slow death of my beloved parents.

All through this we had also to find out if Rod had any brain abnormalities that could lead to an aneurysm. This lead to an MRA scan and subsequent wait for results. It was not entirely conclusive and has to be repeated in the future. More upset and stress. In June 1998 we received a panicky phone call from Mum to say that dad had collapsed with what looked like a heart attack. He was rushed into hospital and I stayed the night with Mum. It was the first time I realised how ill Mum really was. She sat up in the chair all night retching and making dreadful wounded animal sounds. She kept apologising but at times was also aggressive to me, shouting for me to go home because I couldn t do anything to help. I was scared and it was a struggle to remember that the cancer was speaking, not my darling Marmie.

Dad didn t appear to be in danger so I got on with taking charge of Mum. I phoned the Macmillan nurses and pleaded for Mum to be admitted to the hospice for help with breathing and pain. She was taken into hospital because there were no beds immediately in the hospice. There followed visits between two different hospitals to keep them both stocked up with food, drink and clean clothes. We were all beginning to crack up. Mum was transferred to a hospice bed. Dad remained in hospital while the doctors argued back and forth about the diagnosis and all our pre-booked holidays loomed large on the horizon. Sam, you were bewildered and cross much of the time because Daddy had to keep taking you away from me when important things had to be done. We were all suffering but none of us could help each other. Eventually Grandad was sent home with some query over the potassium levels in his body possibly causing the problems. Due to a huge misunderstanding Nan was also discharged home complete with morphine and oxygen, nebulisers and enough drugs to stock an apothecary. We were all astounded that our darling Mum and dad were being sent home to fend for themselves. A nurse was tending to Mum morning and night but at times to suit herself, not my Mum. The drugs resulted in Mum being doubly incontinent, unbeknown to all of us, and dad was coping alone with cleaning her and washing the bed linen. My heart bleeds when I think of him struggling alone with the heavy work. She felt so terrible by that stage that she constantly shouted at dad. It was the morphine, the pain and the fear talking. This awful situation of her being home only lasted two days. Sam, you may have a vague recollection of buying your wooden train set and red-ted and then going to the flat and spending the day playing with the train on the floor next to Nannie s bed. That was the second of those two days and the last full day that Nannie ever spent at home.

The following morning, Saturday, Mum screamed at dad to help her because she was choking for breath. We were all alerted and the GP called. No Macmillan nurse ever came near us throughout any of this time and the GP, although good with Mum, was not particularly interested (understandably I suppose) in what we were going through. Mum was admitted to hospital very late that day. Sam, this was the day that your Auntie took you to see 'Stardog' at the Polka Theatre. You hated that day so much, the show scared you and you again were forcibly wrenched away from us. I had to stay with Nannie and go in the ambulance with her, so I couldn't give you the attention you needed.

The journey to the hospital was touch and go so we had to go steady. Once settled in bed Mum looked more relaxed and started to feel more settled. Rod and I drove home with awful torrential rain outside the car and floods of depressed tears inside the car. Later that evening Mum was told that she couldn't stay indefinitely and soon would have to go home. That was really the start of the nightmare. We were facing numerous problems. We were all torn between our children and taking care of our parents. Mum was fairly delirious on morphine and dad was scared and very aggressive because of the fear. Mum was lucid and acted perfectly normally some of the time but not all of the time. This, sadly, resulted in us having to be wary of everything that she told us. However, in this instance, the nursing staff confirmed that Mum wasn t particularly welcome on the ward because the hospital had handed her care to the hospice. The hospice was full and Mum wasn t considered ill enough to be re-admitted anyway. We were left wondering how ill she was supposed to get. This was the beginning of August. Dad and I were the only two witnesses to the breathless, guttural-sound attacks that Mum suffered and medical staff considered that they were more-or-less panic attacks. It was so confusing and bewildering. Mum was grudgingly accepted back to the hospice on the 5th August 1998, settled in by you, dear Jamie. How much she loved you, and was deeply grateful that you were with her that day. When I visited that evening she wept with joy when she said that you had told her you loved her. You could not have given her a more treasured gift that would stay with her for all time. She and we were told that she could have a week s respite care and then must go home. Dad and I protested that there was no one at home that could nurse Mum, and the implied reply was that normally relatives love their sick ones enough to do it. Mum listened to these conversations with her dear little face visibly crumbling, so I immediately (with trepidation) told Mum that she could come and live with me. Her happiness and gratitude shone out of her face and I thought at last we d found the answer to smoothing her last few months. Dad also asked me quietly to check out some private nursing homes so I began speaking to the social workers at the hospital. I was informed that if Mum lived with me, all nursing help would be withdrawn by the state and that it would be impossible for me to do it. So I started to phone the homes. They sounded uncaring, money grabbing and far too expensive to put Mum in for an indefinite period. In any case, she didn t want to go. Dad and I felt like we were between a rock and hard place and all we wanted to do was lay down and cry. By the Saturday of that week Dad and I were alone because my two sisters were both away on holidays. Ours was due to commence on the 19th August 1998. Dad and I decided that the only course of action was to hope that Mum would be welcome at the hospice until the rest of the family returned so that we could arrive at solutions together to our sad dilemma. I hired a beautiful car to allow me freedom and mobility because I was dad s lifeline as well as Mum s. I was definitely living on adrenaline at that time. I had been granted carer s leave from work for each afternoon that week to collect dad and go to Mum every day. It was sweltering hot that Monday, 10th August as I started my week of working, parenting and caring for dependent parents. I was scared, tired and worried. Dad did everything he could to fend for himself, provided he could rely on me to get him to the hospice for the afternoon. Each morning I would phone Mum and dad would phone Mum, because she d get very weepy if we didn t. Sometimes she didn t know night from day but she d know if we didn t phone. Occasionally when I phoned her she d be crying anyway and would always tell me she loved you both and Rod and I. There was nothing I could do to help her and I would always feel drained and distressed after each call. One day that week when Dad and I were at the hospice with her, Mum was very distressed about never being able to drink coffee. We asked her if she found it too strong. No, she said, she had to constantly search for the fox and never found one. Without a fox she couldn t drink the coffee. The following day I asked about the foxes. Oh, she said, I ve solved the problem. I drink tea now! She was perfectly serious and obviously meant every word, but Dad and I nearly collapsed laughing. The morphine was talking again. On that same afternoon Mum and dad reminisced about their courting days. They laughed, but mostly sobbed. Dad visibly shrunk into helplessness that afternoon and Mum told him that she hadn t meant to shout at him all those times and that she really loved him. He looked like a little boy let loose in a big sweet shop. After telling him that, she turned to me and said, "I don't know what you've been doing lately but you've started to look quite good!" Praise indeed considering I'd worked out four/five times a week in the gym for seven months! Every afternoon I massaged her hands, arms, legs and feet because her circulation was so bad that she was cold and in pain, despite the morphine. Her method of coercing me each day was to say that nurses and doctors had noticed how smooth her skin had become. Cheeky monkey! Her skin hung in folds with sore scaliness, her flesh having been taken by the cancer. But her toe and fingernails remained painted, her lipstick applied and a crochet set at the foot of her bed awaited her attention. She was attempting to produce blankets for other hospice patients. On the Wednesday afternoon, the 12th August, she spent the whole time furiously leafing through all her magazines to find an outfit from a well-known children's retailer that she wanted me to buy for you Sam. It was really horrible but I assured her I would get it for you. I didn t. She also described two outfits that she wanted Dad and I to bring in from her wardrobe, actually telling us exactly where we would find them and what they looked like. She needed clothes to go away in, she said. We were confused but nevertheless decided to comply. I was looking forward to going to work the following morning because it was my last day in before our holiday and my 40th birthday (the 21st). Unfortunately, events dictated a change of plan. Very early that morning dad called me to say he d had a very dizzy, light-headed session and that he d called the GP. I went to work with cakes to celebrate my forthcoming birthday and received cards and presents from my dear colleagues. Neither dad nor I had called Mum that morning due to time constraints and a shift in need. I arranged with my manager to leave work mid-morning to go and be with Dad. I knew Mum was being cared for but Dad needed me. I bid my goodbyes to my colleagues and set off. The GP had been and gone by the time I arrived. He had prescribed some sort of drugs, for placebo effect I am sure, because he'd told Dad that they both knew he wasn't a well man and couldn't expect to feel fine all the time. I set off to the chemist, phoned Rod to put him in the picture and collected Dad's tablets. He had partially found Mum's clothes, so I found the rest and left Dad taking his tablets. He couldn't wait to get to the hospice because he felt guilty about not phoning Mum that morning. As we were securing the front door we heard the telephone ringing. Dad told me to get the clothes to the car and he'd do a ring-back. It was the hospice. We were told to see the nurses prior to going into Mum's room. The journey was awful. The two of us were choked with our own private fears, but each trying to be blasé for the other.

Arrival at the Hospice

As we parked the car, just outside the entrance, there was a second car parked with its people crowded around huddled together and wailing with sorrow. It sent horror through both of us and Dad looked visibly shocked and shaken. He resembled a small child awaiting an unjust punishment. Still, he held his head up and regained his stature, looking patriarchal and smart in his suit and tie.

Dad and I slowly entered the hospice with fear and trepidation unspoken between us.

On the slow walk to the room we passed the physiotherapist to whom Mum had taken an instant dislike. She looked suitably downcast and shrugged at me with empathy. I could have smacked her cheeky face. She had made Mum s life a misery for the past week.

As we approached Mum s room we were met by a nurse whom Mum had held in high esteem. She stopped us and asked us to take a seat on the settee near the windows. As she sat between us and held one of Dad s and one of my hands the terror shot through my spine and a very surreal air surrounded me from that moment on.

An hour previously Mum had been talking to a friend who was visiting and had suddenly held onto her hands and cried that she was very frightened. She immediately became very breathless and her friend had summoned help. Our lovely nurse administered a large dose of morphine that had the effect of easing the breathing and Mum drifted blissfully into a state of coma-like sleep. Her breathing was no longer bothering her. We were told we were nearing the end and if there was any other family reachable then we needed to do it. I dissolved into wracking sobs and held onto Dad who was suddenly a little more composed than I was. We were ushered in where we found Mum s friend distraught and more than grateful to hand over the pain to us. I hugged and thanked her for being with Mum at the moment that for so long had been Mum s fear. Mum s breathing was laboured and noisy and that was the point, I think, that Dad finally accepted the inevitable. His crumpled, crumbling little face held the sorrow of the last four years while he slowly waited for the love of his life to leave him. I immediately used the phone on the bedside table to set about finding my sisters. Those poor girls, having to race home from their holidays.

Eventually they were tracked down and it was arranged that my younger sister would catch the first flight from Jersey and be with us early evening and my elder sister would start the long drive back from the North, hopefully arriving in the early hours of the morning. Dad and I wondered if either of them would make it. Rod took the reins of our family and I settled in a chair next to Mum and held her hand, her arm, massaged her legs and stroked her hair.

At first we talked over Mum, until our nurse arrived to connect a syringe driver to continuously administer enough morphine to control pain, control breathing and allow Mum to comfortably slip into oblivion. As this was carried out the nurse spoke gently to Mum explaining the process all the while. Dad hurriedly asked if Mum could hear us all talking. We were assured that the last sense to fade is the hearing so we were shocked into tailoring the conversation accordingly. I found it difficult and Dad almost impossible to smalltalk under the circumstances, so talk was limited to soft, soothing, loving comments aimed at Mum. Another of Mum s friend s appeared out of the blue to visit and walked straight into the sadness. She was wonderful with her matter-of-fact chat and managed to lift the mood somewhat by describing good times they d had on outings. Suddenly in our imaginary world Mum was laughing and entertaining in the sunshine of my sisters veranda. The mood plummeted when Dad lay across Mum s legs and sobbed, saying that all he could now see in his mind was his nineteen year old lover in her beautiful high heeled shoes and her white coat. It was murderous to witness such a tragic scene.

Dad decided to take advantage of the friends visit and took a taxicab home to get changed, make himself comfortable and take his medicaments. If I m honest I was angry with him silently and thought he wasn t coming back. However, much to my relief and guilt he returned just one hour later in his wheelchair and in more casual clothing. There had been no change at all in Mum thank goodness, so as Mum s friend left, Dad and I settled down to drink tea and wait for the others to arrive.

My younger sister arrived at 7 o clock and she and I clung together like Hansel and Gretal at the entrance to the hospice, crying and rocking in disbelief. I gave her space with Mum and she too flung herself across the bed moaning and sobbing. I waited a while and then took the opportunity to drive the hire car home before I became incapable of driving, and showered and changed into comfortable clothing. I was more than relieved to return an hour later in a cab to discover no change. The events took on an even more surreal feel as the hours went by and nothing changed. Dad was worn out and the nurses helped with toast, drinks, biscuits and painkillers for him. A bed settee was brought in with a duvet and pillows and my sister and I snuggled, even giggled like children again. From time to time we tried to read and do crosswords and occasionally cuddle and comfort Mum. We didn t manage to sleep, but at least we were comfortable. The nurses were very attentive. As Mum s feet and legs got colder and colder I massaged harder and harder to relieve the pain but more because she so loved that sort of contact. Our elder sister arrived in the middle of the night and pressed a silver cross into Mum s hands. It was upsetting and perturbing to hear the deep, rasping, laboured breathing that became a constant background sound that never changed. We didn t want to lose Mum but the lengthiness of each hour as we became tired and irritable became a little hard to bear. We knew at any time that the morphine could be increased and the going hastened but Dad adamantly stated that nature was to take its course. At 7 o clock in the morning we were chased out of the room to allow the nurses to make Mum more comfortable.

There was an enormous change on our return. Mum s skin was sallow, her breathing very shallow and somehow there was already a distance between us. We were told to give her permission to die, which we did and at 7.30am on 14th August 1998 her last, long, almost inaudible breath was taken. We surrounded the bed and just silently cried as we looked at her with grey skin, no glasses and an almost skeletal expression on her face. It wasn t Mum anymore. She had immediately left that useless body that had so prematurely betrayed her.

I didn t feel pain in my conscious being, but distantly I felt despair, exhaustion, weakness and an overwhelming sense of abandonment and I looked Dad for parental comfort and guidance, only to see a crumbled, lost and abandoned man.

What were we all to do? The lynchpin of the family was gone.

Very quickly we took positive action (survival instinct I suppose). We all needed sustenance and Rod and I had to quickly cancel our holiday and re-book some sort of break for the following weekend. Looking back, I now consider this to be fairly bizarre behaviour but we craved, needed and were hungry for normality. Unfortunately our normality as we had known it could never again be reality. Somehow we all got through that week. My younger sister was back (reluctantly) in Jersey with her family, while the rest of us went through the motions of organising Mum s funeral. My house was like a florist that week. A week which celebrated our wedding anniversary and my 40th birthday as well as commiserating our tragic loss. Dad became very spiritual and sang hymns all the time, whilst efficiently tending to legal and financial affairs. He broke down in the florist s whilst organising her wreath. I ordered a large white pillow of flowers, because for so long Mum wasn t able to enjoy the comfort of lying down. Now she could rest comfortably for ever.

The funeral was beautiful and yet unbearable. In that pristine coffin with its highly polished handles was my Mummy. My world, my carer, my leveller, my biggest fan, my love, my life, my "Mummy muddles". We attempted to sing the hymns, the titles of which we had found written in her diary. And because of Dad we held our head's high and respected Mum with the least spectacle.

During the previous week, whilst discussing plans, Dad had made the statement that will forever be in our minds. Some people have a 'do' and some people don't. AND WE DON'T! But of course we had a 'do' held at my younger sister's house and attended by family and close friends. It would have been a lovely 'do' if Mum had been there and it became hard to remember that she wasn't tucked in a corner somewhere enjoying something to eat. It was the 20th August 1998, the eve before my 40th birthday.

We travelled to Menorca that night to our exorbitantly priced one week of self-catered holiday. The distance put an even more unreal slant on the week and I was constantly fighting guilt about leaving Dad and you, Jamie. I spent the entire week scanning every corner of the complex for Mum, because I was so convinced she d come to see me. I was angry at people having a carefree time while the surrealism slipped away leaving raw open pain in its place. I phoned Dad daily and his little distant breaking voice started to eat away at my heart. I couldn t wait for the week to end.

The day after we arrived home we shared our usual Saturday morning breakfast with Dad and he sat with tears spilling down his face as he drank coffee. Sam, you were constantly bewildered and insecure by this stage because you were surrounded by crying people and you were so angry that I wouldn t take you to see Nanny. Your beloved Grandad could not help you at this time and that made you scared as well as angry. We couldn t make you understand and felt so helpless. Dad didn t want to see any of us on the Sunday so we had several phone conversations, which became progressively apathetic. The following day, August Bank Holiday Monday, Dad woke with chest pains and my elder sister was with him when he was admitted to hospital, on the cardiac ward. It s difficult to explain our feelings. My younger sister had to return early from a weekend away and my elder sister and I did the settling in to hospital bit and shopping for various bits of food. Absolutely honestly we were all thoroughly in disbelief. Dad was like a young insecure boy desperate for his Mum to kiss him better. His chest pains were just a symptom of his feelings and probably due to his lack of sleep, and the doctors couldn t find anything wrong. We were all absolutely exhausted and fed up with this latest development.

It was decided to admit him to be safe and we all came home with lists of things to take in the next day. Oh God, here we go again.

It was my first day back into the office the next day, after I had found the exact bread rolls and correct weight of cheese to take to Dad for his breakfast. He looked lonely and small but no one seemed worried, just concerned about his apathy. My colleagues were sympathetic about Mum and looked at me in disbelief when I told them that Dad was in the care of the coronary ward. I had not even started to grieve for Mum yet. I felt like a spoiled child doing something outrageous for attention. The following three days were very strange. Dad was taken into the intensive care coronary ward for symptoms that were never fully explained to us. He seemed an enigma to the numerous consultants involved in his care and depending on whom we spoke to we were given hope or desperation.

On Saturday morning I received a very early morning call to go in quickly to see the consultant. We all went. The Coronary Care consultant told us that Dad was in end stage cardiomyopathy and that his remaining leg had become gangrenous and needed amputating. He could not withstand an anaesthetic and therefore he should be kept pain-free, loved and comfortable. According to the doctor he was literally dying of a broken heart. Two days prior to this Dad had said to all of us, "I'm so sorry girls, but I need to go to see the muds" (a very affectionate term for Mum).

Automatic pilot definitely took over at that stage as we all settled down for a bedside vigil. We were given a side-room, and the Hilton it was not. The curtains didn't fit lengthways or widthways, cracks in the wall were held together by sticking plaster and it was freezing because the window wasn't shut. Dad had only two days to live at the most. We could almost hear Mum complaining about the curtains and in a way it eased the tension. We felt no real pain in those moments, just disbelief, if anything. So we all settled once again, around a bed, but this time there was no adult, no parent, to help us. The nurses were considerate on the Saturday as the hours dragged on. All our men were wonderful keeping the home fires burning for our bewildered children. Dad s hands started to turn black, then his nose, then his wrists. This sounds pretty gruesome but to us it was our darling Daddy who had been loving, caring, nurturing, funny, strict, scary, but above all, always there for us. The patriarch, the rock upon which we stood. And now that rock was eroding into the sea and shaking our very foundations, our meaning of life. We took it in turns to hold his hands because he seemed to remain aware of us throughout. He clung to us as we clung to him. Saturday night came with no change and my younger sister and I went home for a freshen-up and rest. My elder sister wouldn t leave.

We arrived back early in the morning to still no change which was a mixed blessing. We were relieved nothing had happened but we were so tired, beaten down and feeling in a sort of unreal limbo. A nurse advised us later not to leave Dad s bedside for lunch, as the end was imminent. The Dads brought all you children to say goodbye to Grandad and he became conscious enough to say goodbye back but when he saw you Samantha he snarled at me to get you out of there. He didn't want you to see him like that and of course he was right. But in my addled brain I decided you needed to see where he was, due to the fact that you were so angry with me for not taking you to see your beloved Nannie. You couldn't hope to understand death. All you knew was that you requested daily to see your Nan and I wouldn't comply. In fact, the week after Nan died you said to Grandad, "Where's my Nannie, did you leave her at home?" The three of us wept whilst drinking coffee in the café, Grandad was torn in two not being able to help you understand. Nannie called you "Bonner Sam", her little bonus, and you brought laughter back to Grandad's life. He positively lit up when you were around. So all you children went back home with your Dads and we once again settled, with chocolate and newspapers.

Late afternoon on the Sunday we were shouting out crossword clues to one another and Dad surfaced from his morphine induced coma and gave us an answer. He was mentally so strong with a treacherous body that had betrayed him so badly. We laughed and cried and became bemused by the hours that we sat there. We even started to imagine that they d got it wrong and that we were forcing Dad to die when he wasn t ready to. In fact, even with all the medical notes in our possession, confirming the awful inevitability of the ending, we ll never be free from those last thoughts. They do and always will, serve to torture us. Dad choked to death on Sunday night around 9 o clock, whilst we were laughing about a crossword. He went with a struggle and we certainly weren t aware of the angels gently showing him the way as we had with Mum. He choked and spluttered his way into oblivion and so convinced were we that he hadn t died that we turned the spotlight on his face to confirm signs of life. Mum had flown a million miles within seconds, but Dad remained. But we found no sign of life. No parent remained to help us through, just three tiny shivering little girls lost in the wilderness. We went home, carrying with us the picture of a grief-stricken, scared and lonely little man, who had died in hospital pyjamas in a shabby room, whilst his three little girls giggled in a huddle. I can t begin to explain what it felt like leaving first Mum and then Dad to be manhandled by strangers.

The following morning we all returned to the hospital to collect dad s property and the death certificate, only to be informed that a post-mortem was needed. It was the very last straw for my sisters and I and we panicked. Why when dad died in hospital at the point the doctors expected him to, was a post-mortem necessary. Because we had made him die when he wasn t ready. That s why. We were too selfish to summon up more energy to care for him properly. Rod, who works at the hospital, reacted to our distress by flying off to find the consultant for some answers. He discovered that one of the junior doctors had ordered the post-mortem mistakenly and the consultant deemed it unnecessary. The damage was done and we remained in shock.

The look on the Funeral Directors face was a picture and will remain forever. There we all sat, <u>again</u>, three weeks after Mum s funeral and you could see that he was probably expecting a complaint. How he kept his face straight when we requested the same service, different parent, was beyond our comprehension. Even through our crippling grief we saw the funny side.

On 14th September 1998, one calendar month after Mum died, we had a repeat of Mum s funeral, except for one piece of music. On Dad s coffee table we had found he had written a verse from Danny Boy . So that s what we all sang. Heads held high just as Dad would have expected.   We voiced our feelings of guilt to the lovely lady minister who conducted both funerals, and she told us that Dad didn t want life without Mum and he wanted to bequeath us the greatest gift of all, Freedom.

Clearing their flat prior to selling was a painful and exciting trip down memory lane. The cupboards were elastic with bag after bag and box after box of memorabilia emerging from the depths. They could have opened a hypermarket and traded for years in wool, tapestries, bed linen, combs, pens and penknives. We all chose little treasures to take home and cherish. Two of my chosen treasures included a crystal bird and a very decorative set of bathroom porcelain. The former, worth a fair bit of money was accidentally dropped and kicked under the car. The latter, I ve since discovered, was purchased for the grand sum of 87p and has survived unscathed! C est la vie. There was laughter but definitely pain and tears. And more tears.

I m sitting here at work, waiting to hear if my job or a job like it will exist in the new departmental structure (we ve just merged with another large NHS Trust). I m currently on the top of a grade that is considered middle to senior management. We have a management team (the DMT) who are a complete hotchpotch of brilliant and qualified accountants down to supercilious, non-qualified individuals. The DMT, some of whom are less qualified than us, are in their weekly meeting, discussing the way they re going to shape our future. Not our duties, but our entire lives. Decisions taken soundly and calculatingly by most but also defensively, fearing their own positions, by some. Charming.

So childishly I m playing solitaire on the computer and writing this. I m having an introspective day today, probably due to two anti-depressant pills last night instead of one, and a sleepless night on the settee with my darling daughter! I love you two, my children. My pride fills all my heart, and Rod s too. He and I frequently row over how much he s spoiling you, Sam, because you know full-well you ve got him dancing to your tune all the time. He tells me that you re only a baby but you are so much like me that I practically know what you re going to say or do, before you do. And it isn t all the action of a baby! Your intelligence occasionally frightens us and leaves us unsure of the way forward.

Your schooling has put us in a quandary for the moment. For Nanny in Heaven, we put your name down for the private grammar school where your cousin goes and we await the interview in January. Our Health Visitor has also encouraged us in that direction because of your ability. However, my fears are for you emotionally. You constantly need cuddles and reassurance and we love doing that too. We re all very cuddly people, but I m wondering how you will be in a school full of children with super-deluxe brains and emotionally mature beyond their years. This may be incorrect, so we'll have to see. I'd rather just put you in my pocket and take you everywhere with me!

This separation from children bit is terribly hard on Mummies too. When I left you, Jamie, all those years ago in the crèche while I worked in the office at the local hospital, you'd cling on to my knees as I was leaving, shouting "Mummy, don't leave" over and over again. How I ever held down that job I'll never understand, because I'd spend half of my part-time hours in floods and floods of tears. In so many ways though it was easier for me to leave you because I had no choice (financially, we were in deep trouble), but now there is an element of choice and a lot of the time I feel tremendous guilt. Sam, you are full of energy, as bright as a button, and adore other children and in Dad's and my opinion the nursery is extremely beneficial. If this is not your perception, then please forgive me and try to understand. When we collect you from nursery, four days per week, we then all go swimming, to attempt to wear you out some more! You still don t sleep all night because you want company. From the day you were born, Dad and I have taken the nights in turn, otherwise we would have been like zombies. We also take it in turns to prise Jamie out of bed in the mornings. Jamie, you re shattered all the time. You re at college doing your first year at A level and, it would seem, working at the supermarket pretty much the rest of the time. Didn t your contract say 15 hours? I m not sure if you ve ever realised the extent of my pride for you. You have enriched my life beyond words, as has your beautiful sister, and I thank God every day for you. Be proud, be kind but most of all be true to yourselves.

Sam, it s your third birthday next Friday and currently hidden in the shed is a motorised pink and white motorbike, bought by Jamie, Dad and me. How excited will you be with it? We are due to move to our new house on the 5th August and if we don t exchange contracts soon, I ll go mad.

All these things we ve been buying you are dependent on having that big garden. The patio at our old house is way, way too small. Fingers crossed. We ve also bought a new bathroom suite for our en-suite that we may have to use as plant pots in this garden if we don t move into the new house. It will cost us a complete fortune, but will not seem that way to you both at the time you re reading this. We decided to move to sensibly invest my inheritance money and also because Nannie Heaven had numerous dreams where she saw Sam drowning in our pond at our old house. She had a terror of water because her cousin drowned at the age of 21, and constantly warned me about our pond. We actually had no intentions of moving at all and it just sort of happened. Ours was sold in four days and the new one was so close by, and so what we needed, that we always felt Nan and Grandad were the instigators in the whole thing. I miss them so badly. The pain has gone but the aching hasn t. Jamie, you ve been tremendous support over the past year, saying the right things and entertaining Sam when things have been overwhelming. Thank you darling, I knew you were in pain too. They were such a big part of our lives. Holidays with them, help with money, advice and guidance and lots of love. Grandad was always a cantankerous curmudgeon, but such a strength for us. I cannot imagine what your career will be, but if it s in the sciences you ll have put him on the highest cloud. Always treasure his books, they should remain family heirlooms for subsequent budding scientists in the family.

Right darlings, it s time to collect you Sam, have a cuddle and swimming here we come.

Your ever-loving

Mummy

XXX

XXX

1st July 1999

I was shown our new merged departmental structure yesterday. My post, which has until now been one of the senior posts in the department, has suddenly been devalued by most of the other middle-management posts being evaluated to higher salaries than mine, while mine has stayed the same. There are three posts in my department. When I told my line manager that I intended to apply for three of the other posts but not mine she was livid and suggested it was probably time to be looking elsewhere. I feel so hurt and betrayed; all I wanted was a fair hearing but as usual I m not one of the chosen few. I m now in the position of applying for and being turned down for the other three and then being out of work.

For a long time here I thought I wasn t wanted and I had just about turned around my thoughts. So here I am again, feeling as needed as a dose of smallpox. Please forgive me children if I decide to stay at home and live on your inheritance. At least you ll have proper meals and clean clothes again. I m feeling really sad today for loads of reasons. Firstly because of work. Secondly, it s your birthday tomorrow, Sammykins, and your darling Nannie Heaven isn t here with us. She would have cried if she had see you wearing your princess dress (your cousin s bridesmaid dress for my wedding) because you are so divinely beautiful.

I just don t know what I m going to do about work.

Tuesday 13th July 1999

We re still in the thick of all this merger rubbish. All the management team have retained their jobs with or without the appropriate qualifications. What a huge surprise that wasn t! I m in the next wave of interviewees and I m sick of the whole subject. My job in the new structure is one of a handful that still has the same salary whilst the others have increased, thereby giving me the feeling of demotion. There are others to apply for but none attractive enough or feasible to do part-time. I have, therefore, applied for a finance position in a local school. I don t know what move to make really and I m hoping that my mind will be made up for me. The school job will be very family friendly and I think that s what we all need and deserve now. The downside is that it pays next to nothing. Is that important? I can t make up my mind. You see my quandary, kids? The school job pays less than my outgoings. Never mind, let s stop the boring talk.

Sam, it was your birthday party at your Auntie s the day before yesterday and you were in an ecstatic mood. We took some photos of you looking stunningly beautiful in the old bridesmaid dress and we collect them today from the developers. If they look nice, everybody we know will receive a copy for framing. I cried when we put the dress on you, do you remember? By the time that Jamie had finished his lunchtime shift at the supermarket you had changed into civvies, which was a great pity.

I have now lost 10lb on my diet which is marvellous because I m 41 in four weeks and don t want to be the stereotypical fat, forty and frumpy!

Samantha, some advice. Look after your appearance. You have been blessed with beauty and you must keep it going. You must keep fit which will keep your curvy shape and treat your skin as if it were porcelain. Your partner / boyfriend / girlfriend / husband must always be kept admiring you. Perfume, softness, kindness and a glint in your eye is what holds a partners attention.

We re taking you swimming daily, which we hope will train you to stay active all through your life. Exercising regularly and eating well is all you need to retain your beauty.

Enough chatter, I need to do some work now.

Bye, darlings xxxxx

20ᵗʰ July 1999

Hello darlings. Your old Mum again.

Today I m sitting in the office having been told that my interview is on Monday for this place. The infants school position was shortlisted without me! They said I hadn t mentioned children in my application. I assumed my love of children was implicit from my application so I was devastated, from the bottom of my heart. With my line manager leaving in a couple of weeks and having to interview loads of people, (for example four people have applied for my job), she s snowed under with work.

She s not in a good mood.

But I really wish she was staying, I will miss her.

27th July 1999

Well darlings,

I had my interview yesterday for this job and I think it went fairly well. I have to wait until next week to be told the decision but I ve already started the new duties so it s looking good. We move home next Friday, 6th August 1999. Last week I suffered the deepest depression that I couldn t shake off. I ve doubled up each evening on anti-depressants and have started to pick up a bit. I cried a lot for my Mum and dad each evening, I suppose because we re nearly at their first anniversary. I can t bear that I won t see them again.

30th July 1999

Since writing the above, I have been laid low with some awful septic throat infection. I wept like a baby when your Aunt took charge and got me the help I needed. At long last I felt nurtured again. I can t bear orphan status. There is no one to show my trophies to (metaphorically speaking) and no one to assure me that I m doing ok and making the right decisions. I don t think my heart will ever smile again. My face will, but not my heart. I still haven t heard about my job but to be honest I don t think I even care any more. Sorry to be so down darlings, but I m lonely and I don t even know who I am anymore. Did I imagine a happy life with supportive parents?

13th August 1999

Dear Jamie and Samantha

We are now settled in our new house. What a beautiful, lovely, cosy, warm and cosseting house this is too. We moved in one week ago today and two of the bedrooms Jamie have been turned into one for you. Our en-suite bathroom has been completely stripped, awaiting decoration, and the garden will begin to be landscaped on Monday. We all feel very happy and settled already. I was offered my job permanently last Wednesday and I accepted because I don t have any real alternative. I feel fine once away from the place and we are currently on our fortnight s annual leave.

We went to the cemetery today to lay flowers for Mum. Although she died on 14th August it was the 13th that we all sat around the bed expecting her demise. We were still full of feeling this time last year, before the numbing effect of pain set in. I have very recently upped my anti-depressants to two daily from one, because the pain and hopelessness have become very acute. The feelings are so strange. The pain isn t really pain but the most incredible sadness. The realisation that nothing you do can ever make them talk to you again, never see this new house or witness you, Sammy, swimming for another badge and certificate. You achieved your 20 metres last Saturday and I thought of Nannie never seeing you swim.

Very strange things have happened since we moved to really make me believe that Nan and Grandad are here with us and today on our return from the cemetery our front garden was littered with white feathers. My younger sister says that white feathers are sprinkled by angels. I want to believe it, so I will.

14th August 1999
(1st Anniversary Mum dying)

We had guests last night. They got drunk, we stayed sober and they didn t leave until nearly 2 o clock this morning. Short of asking them to leave, Rod did everything he could to persuade them to leave. He locked the house up for the night, I put the game away and cleared the dishes etc but still they lingered. Eventually, just before 2o clock they cleared off. What a nightmare! We are just not party animals. So here we are after three hours sleep wondering what we re supposed to be feeling. I m reliving every minute of the events of a year ago, but then I have been every day anyway. A year ago today was a numb day, trying to believe and accept that Mum had died.

Samantha, my lovely girl, you are currently playing with your cousin, another one of our lovely girls, and the chatter is uplifting. Today I feel strangely grateful for just surviving the year. What a happy, happy house this is. Oh dear God, please let this be a turn of fortune for us all. Yes, there s sufficient money and that can t be understated, but people mean more, much much more than money. I would give everything away to have my people back again.

Well, we re all off swimming now to see if Sam can achieve her 30 metres. I ll sign off and write soon.

Much love

Mum
X X X X

23rd August 1999

Well my beautiful kids, here I am on the first morning of my new job, deputising for the Financial Accountant and trying to teach a new assistant. It s like the deaf and dumb trying to lead the blind and lame! Today, more than ever, I wonder why I m still working. I would much rather have my feet up in front of the telly with a book of puzzles to keep my brain active. Help!!

Anyway, back to reality. Last week, the 20th August, which was the first anniversary of the last day for us to be with Nannie, before her coffin was taken away from us, hit us all like a sledgehammer. I found it harder than the anniversary of the day she died, I think because you still own the person until the funeral. I found it devastating to walk away and leave her, feeling the same way as if walking away and abandoning a helpless lonely child. We knew that day she was gone, whether we could cope or not and nothing could make it better for us. Each day I m reliving this time last year and feeling the same pain and helplessness.

Enough of the sadness.

I m sitting at work trying to look as if I m writing a draft report or something but really daydreaming about what to feed all the family when they come round on Sunday. I have received instructions from my darling sisters to make chocolate pear pudding just the way Mum did, where the marshmallows have to be just the right amount of chewy and the almonds toasted to perfection.

We had the most spectacular day last Sunday when the whole family came to our new home for loads of food. Roast beef and desserts that could sink the QE2!

I love my sisters with all my heart and really need them now like never before. I m horribly jealous of them both of course because they re both so beautiful and so slim. My older sister always looks gorgeous and natural; my younger sister always keeps up with fashion and knows just what suits her. She had her natural hair colour restored and when she walked through the door I swear all the years melted away and she looked like my baby sister again. I felt fat and ugly next to both of them. My younger sister even offered me a facial so she must have thought it too; but nevertheless I was very grateful. The one thing that has faded out of my marriage is the lovely neck and head pampering. Inevitable, I suppose, but I so miss it. The facial was deliciously relaxing.

The second thing I m jealous of is the bond that my sisters share. They always go to each other first before coming to me and the only way I ve learnt to cope with it is to act as though I m not really interested. The alternative is to keep butting in and asking what they re talking about. Not very appealing to me, that option. All my life I ve felt like an outsider, different somehow. I can t explain it any further except I know you, Jamie, feel the same and I get the impression that my second to eldest nephew does too, though I ve never spoken to him about it. How much space in my heart does that boy take up. I can see through all the male macho behaviour and see the golden person with the warmest heart. I think the loss of beloved Nannie has travelled deep within his soul. He had a very special place in Nannie s heart as did all you beloved grandchildren.

I have craved being closed to my sisters the way they are together but that s not to be in this lifetime. I adore, really adore all of you, my husband, my children, my sisters and my nieces and nephews.

Monday 6th September 1999

This is probably one of the lowest days of my entire life so far.

I m ashamed of my writings of the 1st September about my jealousy for my sisters.

Last night I started off shivering uncontrollably and ended up by being drenched in perspiration. Apart from it being the first anniversary of Dad dying, I also feel as though I m becoming fairly seriously ill. Shock has always affected me this way. Already my voice is starting to fade. I feel like a tiny abandoned child in a huge bare room where there s nowhere to hide and no one to hold. I dreamt last night of my Aunts (still very alive) funeral followed by us buying a summer home on a mobile home park?! The funeral was very distressing because the music was the same as Mum and Dad s. Make me a channel of your peace. This morning I woke up and I could not believe it is all true. It s as if I haven t acknowledged the loss of Mum and

Dad before. They re never coming back and I can t bear it. That s a statement we all make daily but until you really feel it you don t realise the abuse of the words. I can t bear it , means you really can t imagine how you can live through each day with the reality. I hope my Aunt is OK. The dream came out of the blue. I think (I hope) that she s not even ill.

I love my sisters as much as I love you, my children, Jamie and Samantha. I want to protect them and take away their pain, but of course I can t. I pray that Mum and Dad are now our guardian angels and have them wrapped in their warm wings. We are the luckiest sisters alive in our husbands and children. Everyone is so supportive, and without the deep love between us and the men, I don t think we could survive. Samantha, you ve been extremely insecure this last weekend because you are so tied up in my emotions that you know something is drastically wrong. I really try, but don t manage, to be ok for you, and I m so sorry darling that I make you fearful.

Throughout the last twenty three months or so (it still feels like yesterday since I lost my parents) I have largely got on with my life, moved into our beautiful new house, spoilt my children with gifts and changed my job.

I eventually moved to a primary school and what an awful culture shock! I knew immediately that I had made a huge mistake. I had gone from a huge establishment where I had spent ten years getting to know and love practically everyone to a very small primary school, where the handful of staff held me at arms length and viewed me with a degree of suspicion. I was still vulnerable and found the people equally if not more dysfunctional than I was. The office was a complete mess with outstanding work dating back several months and an absolute hands-off attitude from staff that I considered could or should be involved. I made one very good friend there though who helped all she could and became a staunch ally throughout. She was

my saviour and the reason I stayed and
battled.

I did all I could to straighten the work and
become a valued Accountant for the school,
despite the crippling loneliness I felt.

The dreams

All my frequent and disturbing dreams
have centred around Mum coming back to
us, unaware that she has already died. My
sisters and I have all dreamt similarly and
sometimes on the same nights. Last night,
for the first time, I dreamt of Dad. I dreamt
he had originally been alive when buried,
so we set about freeing him. This wasn t in
the least bit scary or macabre in the dream,
but we all felt guilt-ridden. I dreamt he was
repeating his illness in coronary care. I was
completely alone with the knowledge of his
illness and didn t believe or understand the
severity. Instead of visiting Dad, I went to
see a hospital doctor and was greeted by
three of the Consultants. The only female
assured me of the gravity of the illness and
told me to repeat this to Dad. YOU NEED

TO LAY YOUR JACKET AT THE ENTRANCE TO THE PEARLY GATES TO ENSURE YOURSELF A PLACE . And she said to me, Whether he wants to or not, or you want him to or not, your Dad will die this time from this illness. There is nothing we can do to stop it . In fear and dread I traipsed round the hospital searching for the coronary care wing and finally found Dad. At that point my elder sister joined me. I didn t need to discuss any of the details with Dad because he said to us as soon as we arrived, Don t worry lovey. I know I m going to die and I m ok with it. I just didn t understand last time. Now I m ready to go . He was calm and genuinely smiling and died very peacefully. For so long we felt as though we had killed him.

The dreams have always centred around the fact that both Mum and Dad come back to life. Only to find that we have sold their home and all their money and belongings have gone in various directions. We have always felt that Dad was lost somewhere in limbo.

This dream was therefore, understandably, amazingly uplifting. When I woke up this morning I instantly felt better and believe Dad is out of purgatory and in heaven.

September 2000

This was when you started your new school, Sam. A wonderful and homely preparatory school we decided on as the alternative when your interview for the large private grammar school went very badly. You were three years old at the time of that interview and part of the test was for you to walk away with a teacher into another room and not look back to Daddy and I for help. You screamed and shouted and cried for us to come to you.

According to a child psychologist from whom I had previously sought advice regarding your regressive behaviour, you were suffering severe separation anxiety. At the age of two, a child begins to learn that when a loved one leaves they always come back. In your case, at the age of two, your beloved Nannie and Grandad, who were almost as large a part of your life as we were, went away and never came back. You lost your learnt security.

You were deemed an unsuitable candidate for the large impersonal school but only after we had decided the school was unsuitable for you.

You were so happy with your new friends and your cosy environment and Daddy and I breathed a sigh of relief.

March/April 2001

We have the results of your needle biopsy, Carolyn. Is there someone you can bring with you to the hospital?

The voice of the doctor on the other end of the phone faded into the distance as my very core filled once again with fear, pain and dread. I knew, I just knew, from the moment I found the lump and skin puckering in my left breast, that I too had cancer. I felt no self-pity, just disbelief, bemusement even. The exhaustion was overwhelming, yet another massive fight ahead of me. It was then, more than ever, that I wished I was still with my old colleagues at the hospital. My new colleagues at the school never knew the old me. I craved familiarity from the people I had worked with and loved for so long, friends who would and could have given me more strength. Needing so much time off in my new post I was viewed as someone who let down the running of the establishment. There was little love and no support. I let them down.

My first operation, a lumpectomy, showed a rapidly growing, fairly highly graded carcinoma that necessitated a radical mastectomy within four weeks, or a very limited prognosis.

My option for immediate reconstruction using back muscle and tissue was to be carried out at the same time as the mastectomy.

So, on the 21st May 2001 I embarked on a gruelling five-hour operation.

I felt so lonely.

I needed my Mum and Dad.

25th May 2001

This is day four, post surgery. The pain has yet to be properly controlled, but perhaps the idea is not to be pain-free. I ve been up and about for the last two days out of sheer bloody-mindedness and the horror of being reliant on someone else.

The operation seemed to have taken much longer than expected and I still don t know why, but I do know I went into theatre with a chest infection that I omitted to mention. The cancer was eating me alive so I would rather have died from anaesthesia than postpone the breast removal. The pain and discomfort is such that I could never have been prepared for it. I had a morphine patient controlled button to press, which was as useful as a cat aspirin. They switched to morphine injections, which gave me some measure of pain-relief but also delirium. The night following my operation I lay flat on my back, unable to move, hardly able to breathe and stared at the ceiling until 5am. No one came to me.

At that point I realised that it was only me that was going to ease things. I somehow had to get out of the lay back position in order to breathe but the slightest move sent hundreds of stabbing pains through my back and ribs.

As breakfast arrived I forced myself up to the edge of the bed and clung shakily to my table. The pain was almost unbearable but I d done it. I persuaded the consultant to take me off morphine and give me dihydrocodeine tablets, an old faithful that I knew would work, and from that moment I knew that only I could get me out of here.

I quickly realise that my two to three stones of extra weight I am carrying is now no longer an issue of vanity but of my health and comfort. My new reconstructed breast is large, tight and high and feels like a clamp. To an asthmatic person like me that is a tortuous feeling, adding to the ever present sensation of partial suffocation.

The little button port (used to control the size of the new breast) that is implanted under my skin is fighting for space amongst the fat and because I m barrel-chested thanks to so many childhood asthma attacks, is now also rubbing against my ribs. There just isn t the space for everything, so the fat has to go. I have also been told by the physiotherapist that carrying extra weight greatly increases the chances of lymphodoema (big arm). End of debate. THE FAT HAS TO GO!

I m in a ward with three other ladies who are fairly elderly and bedridden. A crude side of me thinks of it as death row. This feeling is further compounded by the frequent visits from the hospital chaplain who appears uninvited at the end of my bed and hands me leaflets highlighting how to tell the children that I might die. As I sit propped up in bed preening and titivating, the snoring from the other inmates echoes through the air. Hypnotic if I m pain-free, aggravating if I m not. The lady next to me, an elderly Indian who is very obviously the typical matriarch of her family, speaks no English but very easily and persistently gets everything her way by clicking fingers, clapping hands and gesturing generally. The television stays off because she doesn t like it. We all swelter in the heat because she doesn t like the window open. And so it goes on. The sweet lady opposite me looks as though she could have already spent a day or two back with her maker and just puts in very brief appearances back with us. Bless her.

It s all too close to death for me to deal with, so I just need to get out!

For some reason I thought they would let me home today. I ve still got three of the five drains in, so had no good reason, but now I know it s going to be another three or four days I feel terribly down. It s the aloneness that s difficult. I know people love me, adore me, support me, but I m doing this on my own. I m sitting in the day room, hearing an old Rod Stewart track and barely able to stop the tears from spilling down my face. I yearn for my lost youth. I certainly didn t realise then that they were the good times.

I need Rod and Sam and Jamie now, so badly. I feel as though I ve been punished and now I feel like I ll be punished more for complaining.

Sam wouldn t cuddle me today. She s so cross each day to come in and go home without me. Of course I understand her actions but it s made me so upset. Her and I have this bond. The uncut umbilical cord. But it s stretching, thinner and thinner.

Please, baby girl, come back to me. Call me momma again. Tell me you love me.

Sorry, self-pity isn t attractive is it?

I love you darlings.

Day six, post-operative. Still here, but not as depressed. I m allowed to go home today for a few hours if I m a good girl and as long as I come back tonight. And tomorrow I m allowed out all day and return in the evening. My weight is going well. I m disciplining myself to three light meals a day and no rubbish, and must have lost a few pounds already.

Well, I ve just been weighed and have lost 3.5kg (nearly 8lbs!) Fabulous, what a good start. Must continue when I go home. No more Ben and Jerry s for me!

Well, I ve just returned from a couple of hours at my younger sisters and I spent the majority of the time crying. Feeling sorry for myself; frightened of bad results on Friday; of dying prematurely, but most of all of breaking my baby s heart. My Sam is so brave and my heart bleeds with love for her. I just want to be able to assure her that I will come home sometime this decade and that I will still be her Mummy.

Please let me go home.

Please let me know my results.

Please let them be really good.

I ll behave, honestly.

Day seven post-operative. Now 4.4kg down (nearly 10lbs). Wonderful.

I came home on day eight.

Being an hormonal tumour I was treated with endocrine rather than chemical therapy following my surgery. I was also prescribed painkillers for pain in my back and bones; sleeping tablets; antidepressants; and various vitamins. My growing tolerance to the morphine-based painkillers resulted in an ever-increasing need.

2002

I ve been attending the hospital for check-ups for the last few months and had another operation. On the 18th January a lot of excess tissue was removed as well as the port. I suffered from a post-operative infection and took ages to recover. None of my lymph nodes showed evidence of cancer spread and I am now considered to be in remission.

Before diagnosis, apart from an obvious hormonal imbalance, (I thought I could be pregnant), prior to finding the lump, I had not been feeling particularly ill. Following the surgeries I never felt well. I fought one illness after another.

A deep-vein thrombosis travelled from my calf to my lung, thankfully dispersing, but leaving a horrible infection in its place.

I felt constantly nauseous especially when I had to take iron tablets for an iron-deficiency.

My body was always swollen from goodness knows what drug.

Both my eyes were affected by severe corneal ulceration causing pain and temporary loss of sight for a few months.
Having given up smoking twenty-two years ago, I started again last week! Today, however, I feel like my lungs are coated in toffee and I am really struggling to breathe. I ve purchased some nicotine gum. It s disgusting!

As gathered from the cigarettes, emotionally I m not marvellous. I take my prescribed painkillers too quickly, then withdraw for a week, scrabbling around looking for over the counter remedies to deal with the pain and withdrawal symptoms.

Despite my (fairly well) outward appearance I know that in a year or so I will be very ill. Since losing Faye and Mike (friends) so suddenly to cancer, my positive attitude has taken a nose dive. I m ashamed for feeling this way and try to fight it but my world feels quite black most of the time. I question the whole living business and struggle to see the point.

My tiredness and apathy grow daily. I find it increasingly hard to go to work and increasingly hard to do anything in the house; and eventually have to give up everything completely by Christmas 2002.

January – September 2003

All the numerous drugs I am ingesting give me a wonderful coping mechanism. A way of dealing with the physical pain but also a way of living on a much lower mental echelon where no pain or hurt can reach. I merely exist, not live, in a thought-free bubble that nothing can penetrate. A form of self-induced breakdown.

I feel like a nobody.

I am a nobody.

I m sinking deeper and deeper into despair.

I need to rest.

I am slowly but surely dying.

11th September 2003

(The second anniversary of that terrible World Trade Centre terrorist day. The day we also lost Faye to oblivion – September 11th 2001)

I have just seen a book I bought but have yet to read, entitled, "I have lived a thousand years", by Livia Bitton-Jackson. Dear God, that is exactly how I feel today.

By accident, decision or whatever other forces are at work, I have, this week, been "detoxing" my brain from the plethora of drugs that I have been living on for the past two years.

Everyone had died.

My beloved parents. My sweet and funny brother-in-law. My newly made hospital friends. (In particular Heather, who showed bravery beyond my comprehension. An inspiration for all of us who knew her). Faye, a dear friend who adored and was adored by her husband and two very young daughters. Mike, a friend s loving husband. All gone. So why would or should *I* be the one to survive. I was gradually buying into the idea that there were no options left open to me, but death. So I sat and waited for God; with my brain numbed with all the drugs available to a cancer patient, wallowing in egocentricity and congratulating myself on being so brave in my dying months. Blissful ignorance, you d think? I, personally, had been anaesthetised against the worst of the pain but my family had watched me sit, unable to move, incapable of being anything other than a vision in the corner of the living room. With visible and tangible misery on their faces, I hazily saw them witness my slow decline into complete uselessness. Kind and gentle comments were made but I had gone too far away. I was unreachable. They sat helpless as I ruined all our lovely possessions with cigarette burns. My son quickly extinguished a fire accidentally started in the lounge, and finally my husband cried the time I hit my head as I fell to my potential death in the bathroom. Feeling no wrong, and seeing no wrong. Taking and scrabbling for more and more comforting tablets and finally encountering a very stupid and misguided (or maybe just caring) locum doctor, who, by feeding me a cocktail of drugs that my system rejected, has finally led me to this path of consciousness and awareness.

I wasn t dying.

I was killing myself, with fear and depression and my family had to watch.

So here I am on my *"Journey Back to the Light."*

Four days ago, it feels like four years, my seven-year-old daughter asked me how she could find the orphanage. What number bus could take her there? How much was the bus fare? Where would she get the fare? Could she find the orphanage by walking? What would she say when she got there? The questions went on and on. What could I say or do with questions like that? I hugged her and told her there would never be a time when any of that was necessary and the utter despair threatened to overwhelm me. What dreadful fear and sadness that little person must be living with. She has seen too much and experienced too much loss in her little lifetime. We have to put it right. *I* have to put it right.

Despite the mental hurt and fear, clarity of mind is the only way I can return to normal. Clarity brings reality and reality can be dealt with. (I have chosen skin patches and deep breathing relaxation, so I can largely ignore my physical pain).

I am thoroughly disgusted to realise I am smoking again. Yet another hurdle to cross for the second time in my life. I kicked that filthy weed twenty-three years ago, for the first time. Now, yet again, I have to do it again. I *cannot* be a smoker. It s revolting, dirty and hardly the path back from cancer. I am repulsed to be sitting in a smoke-filled house, knowing that this is the atmosphere that my family live in. Why have I never seem smelt or felt this before now? My poor baby girl coughs, sneezes and splutters her way through the days and it s been my fault. Loving and nurturing? I don t think so. But please don t misunderstand. I don t blame myself entirely. I have been in a deep, dark place. Sucked into a vortex of grief, pain, fear, near death and painkilling drugs too strong to handle. I also fell between help at the hospital. Many trials were carried out; relaxation and stress-reduction type trials that I was not eligible for because I am too young! This is not a complaint of the wonderful hospital but just an example of the difficulties I encountered.

The practical stuff can be dealt with as my strength grows day by day. I'll give up the cigarettes. I'll clean the house. I'll nurture my children. I truly will. These last few days have been absolutely the worst of my entire life and I could never relive them again.

Five years ago, the loss of my beloved parents. A devastating loss indescribable in its' depths and the associated feelings of guilt.

Two weeks after Mum died, when I had no more left to give, I felt anger that Dad suddenly had to grab the limelight, and squeeze more and more from us. How were we to know he too was dying? Had we willed it? (That question tortured me then and tortures me still). We were so tired and needed love and nurture, not another very needy person. So we continued to care – repressing anger, stifling grief – another funeral – sorting possessions. Three little girls sitting catapulted and orphaned in Mummy and

Daddy s house. Opening private drawers and cupboards previously forbidden, unravelling their lives and love. Adult women, but three such despairing and lost children.

To then learn that I too had cancer. Was I relieved? Was I grateful for the perceived punishment for feeling anger and exhaustion at other people s continuous demands? Did I see it as a way to be with Mum and Dad again? Or did I just see a path of restfulness and caring? I had no more resources left to give to my family, so why not just slip quietly away? But after radical surgery maybe the cancer went. Maybe it s gone. Maybe it will never come back.

Yet, after all that, yes, these few days have been the worst of my life. Lying alone physically and emotionally, watching every second tick away on the clock, day and night. Feeling the comfort of the drugs seeping away from the nerves, vessels, and corners of my battered body and brain.

Unravelling, re-awakening areas of the consciousness previously shut down, blotted out, away from pain too difficult to see. To be replaced by real physical, tangible pain. Vice-like pain throughout my back and chest, gripping, stabbing, but come now. Relax, breathe slowly, breathe, relax. But my mind. Is there pain? Is there sorrow? I honestly feel devoid of pain in my mind. Instead there is calmness, a peace, a realisation that it has gone. The pain, the guilt, the feelings of inadequacies, of not giving enough, of being a taker. I know in the depths of my soul that I have never taken. Just given and given some more, until there was nothing left to give. My beautiful, strong and loving parents were just tired people too. I wanted and needed more but they just had nothing left.

(Detoxification   My   own   experience
(COLD TURKEY))

You are a computer, and you come with an operating system. We ll call that **'ME'**.

A different system, **'MORPHINE'** runs you better, faster, but needs constant and increasing input . Input is suddenly withdrawn and **'MORPHINE'** walks out, laughing. For an instant there is nothing. Dark, black, lifeless, eternal void. The default system, **'ME'** recognises failure and tries to waken. **'ME'**, furiously and perilously scans cells and vessels for signs of previous unaided activity. Nothing but scrambled code and viruses now not understood. Complete shutdown whilst **'ME'** starts from scratch, unscrambling, decoding, slowly, tired, mending cracks, eradicating forgotten viruses. Power supply only just strong enough to run **ME'** but not the peripherals. **'ME'** rests, just surviving shutdown. Strength building,

ME starts to recover and realises it s job was to lead the others. The thin light from the torch shines down each corridor. Signs of life? No, I ll come back. Hurry on to the next. This one is fine. But conserve energy. Off goes the torch. Oh God, this one needs help. **ME** struggles as other survivors are calling thinly for help. There is only me, so wait and I ll be there. Please be patient. The one I found fine feels abandoned and cries. **ME** reassures loudly. You will be ok, I ll be back, I promise. I have to save all of us. **MORPHINE** laughs loudly from afar. *You can't do it!* come the taunts. **ME** can only ignore it, just enough energy to survive, not follow, not reply. Rest, must rest. Firstly back to the one that was fine. The cries have stopped, resolve has picked up and another torch is found. More help. Thank God. Doors are locked, slammed shut, rusted over. Wait, I hear something in that room. **ME** pulls, pushes and kicks weakly at the solid door. It s stuck. Won t budge. Too tired, must rest, just rest. Refreshed and fed **ME** tries again. This time success. More light and more help.

The weak ones will be returned to. **ME** knows there is life. Off goes the torch. Batteries are weak and **ME** has no recollection of the old supply. But wait, **ME** is rechargeable, plug in and wait for strength. Lights flicker, fade, grow, then remain on. More and more light. **ME** breathes a sigh of relief, **ME** shouts to **MORPHINE**, You were too fancy, too needy, too expensive. *High Maintenance.* You re not needed here . **ME** is back. Rest, conserve energy, rest, **ME** is in control. Older, tired, but back. No cost, no requirements, no support. Just dependable **ME** .

To translate this detoxification process it is important to understand that it takes weeks for the body to function properly. Some days vision is fine and later days it shuts down to allow the body the strength to regain other functions. This applies to walking and fine motor skills of the hands and every function and every sense is affected. Some days I couldn t focus at all, other days everything loomed large in technicolour and was actually quite frightening. My hearing fluctuated between near-deafness and piercing pain, even from the sound of a bird tweeting. If I stood up my feet would become numb and walking was sometimes near impossible. The sense of smell became so acute one day that even beautiful previously adored aftershave and perfume caused acute nausea. I know I will never be able again to accept those fragrances without recalling the horror of detoxification. I had no feelings in my fingers for the longest time which served to hamper almost everything I tried to do.

Obviously, to go through this process it would be ideal and probably safer to be in a rehabilitation unit, with people at your beck and call, and counsellors and fellow sufferers; but I am too private and wanted no more time away from my family. I needed to be chemical-free and allow my brain to find the normal settings of my body as quickly and as safely as was possible. Right or wrong, I ve done it.

The hardest I felt to deal with was the awful disorientation and light-headedness that seemed to last forever. I never imagined I could again produce a meal for my family, drive a car, or even stand up for considerable periods of time. The only way through is to rest, eat sensibly (I lost four stones in this process) and be kind to yourself. Each day you feel different. Not necessarily better, but different. I had one day, after two weeks, of complete and utter euphoria. I suppose my body must have been resetting the dopamine levels, but whatever it was I could have bottled it and become a millionaire. I was distraught when I woke up the next day feeling flat.

Some days can be very difficult when it seems easier to resort to drugs to take away the pain and reality; because reality isn t all it s cracked up to be. Right? Wrong. So many days have gone past, so much hard work done. The path now being travelled is honest and the mind is clear.

I have been left with some disabilities from my cancer. For example, I very nearly lost my eyesight earlier this year, but timely intervention saved one eye completely and has left me only partial scarring in the other. I have scars and pain in my back but also, if I m allowed to show off a little, a cleavage to die for. I have a figure I have always craved and fully intend to keep it by eating sensibly and sleeping properly, which is something I had lost along the way. Some weeks I would only sleep for a couple of hours and days would pass before I remembered to eat. My skin glows now where it was grey before and I look alive. Numerous people have commented that I look ten years younger than my real age of forty-five and a hundred years younger than I did a few weeks ago! I am still limited in energy and have no idea if or how long I will remain in remission from breast cancer.

I have been in a carefree world where my mind and soul were healing, so perhaps the journey was very necessary. Who knows? I would love to claim complete insight but I have more questions than answers.

However, I do know one thing for sure. I can now fight using my mind, where my ultimate strength can be found.

I am determined never again to fall into the abyss.

THE END